Borderline Personality Disorder Guidance

Living With & Understanding This Condition

By Peter Kornfeld
Copyright © 2013

Income Disclaimer

This book contains business strategies, marketing methods and other business advice that, regardless of my own results and experience, may not produce the same results (or any results) for you. I make absolutely no guarantee, expressed or implied, that by following the advice below you will make any money or improve current profits, as there are several factors and variables that come into play regarding any given business.

Primarily, results will depend on the nature of the product or business model, the conditions of the marketplace, the experience of the individual, and situations and elements that are beyond your control.

As with any business endeavor, you assume all risk related to investment and money based on your own discretion and at your own potential expense.

Liability Disclaimer

By reading this book, you assume all risks associated with using the advice given below, with a full understanding that you, solely, are responsible for anything that may occur as a result of putting this information into action in any way, and regardless of your interpretation of the advice.

You further agree that our company cannot be held responsible in any way for the success or failure of your business as a result of the information presented in this book. It is your responsibility to conduct your own due diligence regarding the safe and successful operation of your business if you intend to apply any of our information in any way to your business operations.

Terms of Use

You are given a non-transferable, "personal use" license to this book. You cannot distribute it or share it with other individuals.

Also, there are no resale rights or private label rights granted when purchasing this book. In other words, it's for your own personal use only.

Borderline Personality Disorder Guidance

Living With & Understanding This Condition

By Peter Kornfeld

Table of Contents

Introduction

There is much about mental health that we as a society don't fully comprehend. Though we may feel that there is a good handle on the most common conditions such as depression, there are many areas that we still need a great deal more insight. One such condition that is often misunderstood misdiagnosed, and therefore difficult to live with is Borderline Personality Disorders.

The truth is that the conditions within this spectrum cover a wide range of variances, and therefore help is truly needed. Though there has been much research and work done to help understand true and deep personality disorders, those who fall within certain areas of the spectrum are left untreated and therefore misunderstood.

A Very Real and Often Misunderstood Medical Condition for All
For the people who suffer from Borderline Personality Disorders (BPD) this can be a lifelong debilitating and very frustrating medical condition. Since the spectrum is so wide, even experts can ignore or brush off the most common symptoms. Sometimes this is confused with other disorders and in some cases it is even brushed off as an unsavory personality overall.

The people who do suffer through BPD in their lives are dealing with very real symptoms that are very difficult to master. They may have a hard time socializing or even functioning in daily life. They may find it difficult to manage relationships or the simple tasks that so many of us take for granted.

This condition and the wide variance that it covers is not just difficult for the individuals who suffer from it, but also for those that are close to them. Family members and close friends who care for those with a BPD may find it very challenging to communicate or to get close to the person suffering from it. Though they may care deeply, they may feel unsure of how to handle the very commonly described cycle of "walking on eggshells".

The key to any sort of Borderline Personality Disorder is to receive a proper diagnosis. Since there is much to be learned about this condition, it is imperative to seek out treatment and perhaps incorporate a second opinion if necessary. Some experts may not fully understand it or the types of symptoms that are closely linked to this mental health condition.

Proper Treatment Can Really Help and Unveil a Path to a Normal and Healthy Life
This is nothing to be taken lightly and the people affected truly need help. This is not an unsavory personality nor is it an individual who just has a hard time getting close to others. This is a legitimate and very frustrating disorder that should be taken seriously and for which treatment should be sought out for as quickly as possible.

The truth is that some individuals who suffer from this condition may not even be aware of it. Just as wide on the spectrum of how this condition is diagnosed are the types and severity of symptoms that may be associated with it. Any unusual behavior accompanied by other symptoms is something to be evaluated by a healthcare professional.

What helps to know, is that there is help for those who suffer from Borderline Personality Disorder. Though much insight can still be gained on this condition, we know much more than we did years ago. For those that can get in touch with the right medical professionals, there is help that can make life feel normal and healthy again.

We will highlight the most common symptoms, treatments, and help the individuals and those close to them understand what this is all about. Sometimes simply seeing what a typical day is like for somebody with a BPD can be rather eye opening. This book is here to help anybody associated with this condition and to provide insight and a path towards treatment.

Before it becomes unbearable for the people that suffer with them, it's time to help those with Borderline Personality Disorders. It's time to highlight this condition, get people the help that they need, and help to restore a bit of normalcy into the process. This can be a livable condition, and with the right help it will be manageable and allow for a normal and healthy life.

What Is Borderline Personality Disorder and How Is It Diagnosed?

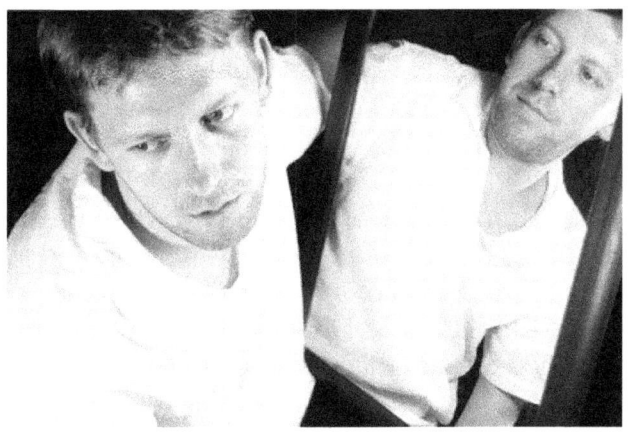

The most important thing to know about borderline personality disorders is that diagnosis is the key. By virtue of the name itself, this is a borderline type of disorder and for that it means that it can be a very gray area. Many health experts may find that they are puzzled because the whole notion of this disorder is newer and therefore quite confusing.

This can be a very disheartening and often frustrating mental health issue for individuals to deal with. Much of that frustration is due to the fact that proper diagnosis can sometimes be hard to find. If you are right on the edge of personality disorder or suffer from other mental health problems, BPD can often be confused with something else. This can mean long term frustration—but there is also much more education and therefore help to be found as well!

Better Comprehension Means More Help For Those Suffering From This
This is not a new disorder, but one of which is becoming more understood and discussed in the mainstream. Many of the symptoms may be confused with depression or other mental health conditions and so it's a sort of an unusual area that many work to understand. Above all, this is something for which the individual suffering from it, should talk to a medical professional if they are at all concerned.

At the core, Borderline Personality Disorder is a mental health disorder that creates significant highs and lows. At the core is a great deal of instability that surfaces primarily within the emotional well being of the victim. It is felt most notably as a mental condition, but as you can imagine it can result in a lot of behavioral issues, acting out, stressful living condition, stress to loved ones close to the victim, and of course a lot of emotional consequences.

People who suffer from BPD often suffer with self esteem issues and may feel worthless or damaged. They may get angry, struggle to develop relationships, be more of a loner or introverted in nature, or simply find it hard to deal with everyday stress. No matter what, it is very obvious that somebody with this type of disorder has some challenges above and beyond other emotional issues in life.

So What Can An Individual With BPD Do To Move Forward?
Sometimes telling the difference between depression, anxiety disorders, and any other slew of mental health conditions can be challenging at best. Many symptoms cross over and it's all about frequency and severity that the individual suffers from. You may ask yourself how exactly something that holds the name "borderline" can

really and truly be diagnosed properly—and it is difficult at times.

The good news for those who suffer from Borderline Personality Disorders is that there is a list of criteria that can be used as a sort of checklist. The standing rule to consider is that if you suffer from five or more of these issues or conditions, then there is a good chance that it is BPD that you suffer from. So understanding what the common symptoms are, is a surefire way to get the help that you so desperately need. We will go through the most common symptoms next to help uncover what may lead to proper treatment.

Diagnosis for BPD comes through a series of tests that a healthcare professional may administer. This may start with a simple consultation to discuss the symptoms and the way in which the person is struggling. From there, psychological evaluation will come next whereby the individual will be observed to see these symptoms in everyday life. This information will be vital in diagnosing and then helping to create a path towards treatment.

There are a number of tests that can be run, but the clinical observation will be the most important first step in the process. Discussing common symptoms, the way that the individual lives their everyday life, and a great deal of discussion will be instrumental in coming up with a proper diagnosis. As more and more healthcare providers are tuning into the common occurrence of BPD, they are being trained to look for symptoms and to get a diagnosis established earlier on in the process than ever before.

Common Symptoms or Signals of This Disorder

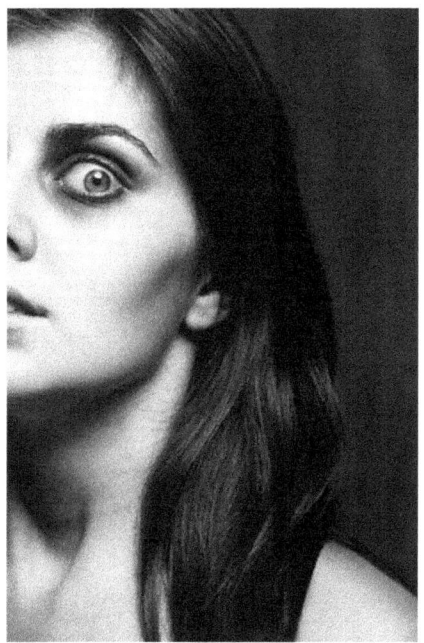

So how can a healthcare professional be sure that it is BPD and not something else? How can an individual hope to get the help that they need or be certain that they even need help in the first place? How can you be sure that it is BPD that is present and not just stress or anxiety present in the individual's life? The good news is that there are some very obvious and telltale symptoms that can help in diagnosing and then treating BPD.
As mentioned, many healthcare professionals will look to see what is happening with the person in their daily life. If

they use a checklist like the one found below to help the diagnosis, then they will be looking for the presence of five of more of these common symptoms. Every case is of course different, but this checklist of symptoms shows very common behavior and therefore works to uncover the truth here.

Some of the most common symptoms of Borderline Personality Disorder are important to understand and they include:

- A pattern and frequency of unstable and sometimes destructive relationships

- Impulsive and often self destructive behaviors that make no sense or tie to no traumatic event—no rhyme or reason for these decisions

- An intense fear of being abandoned or being alone, which may stem from something more serious or stand alone as a symptom

- Feeling intensely bad about yourself to the point where there may be harmful behavior or the feeling of hopelessness or self hatred

- Very wild mood swings—high highs to low lows with no real middle ground in between that leaves the individual mentally exhausted

- Feeling empty, hollow, or nothing inside no matter what else may be going on in life

- Injuring yourself or having the intent to do so, with the extreme being suicidal behavior or attempts

- Anger management issues that are extreme in nature and may result in physical damage to oneself, to others, or to a property

- Paranoia in an extreme sense that keeps the individual from attaching to everyday life and reality

- An unrealistic and often harmful view of yourself, of relationships, or of the world which can be harmful and sometimes dangerous

- Having a very difficult time in functioning in everyday life, in holding down a job, in developing or holding onto relationships, or to handling simple daily activities

Some of these are very extreme in nature and some are more minor and can therefore be confused with other things. These are not usually subtle symptoms, but the frequency they are suffering and the severity may vary by individual. This checklist can be of great help to an individual who suspects BPD or to a health care professional who is trying to uncover and therefore diagnose it.

Though it may be initially confused with something else, it becomes quite evident when there is the presence of multiple symptoms that something is amiss. Though "borderline" may be deceptive in nature, it all makes sense after a while. Sometimes the individual may function okay in everyday life, but then runs into these roadblocks from time to time that make "normal" life nearly impossible. Simply understanding these symptoms can be of great help in allowing an individual to move forward with their life!

Causes of Borderline Personality Disorder

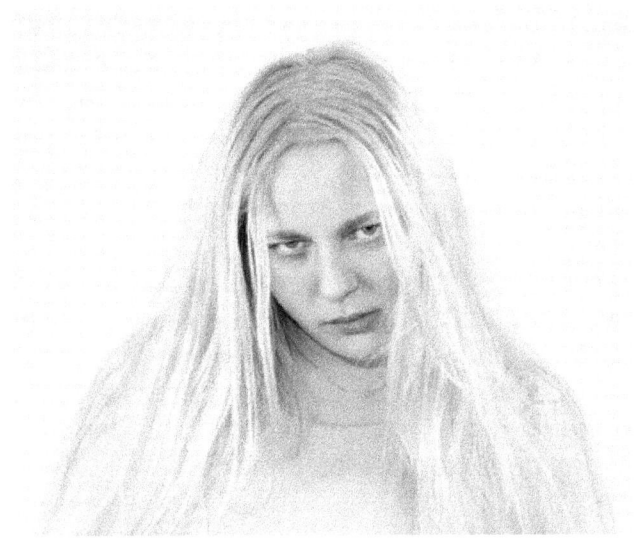

For those that suffer from Borderline Personality Disorder, the question always comes up as to what causes it? Even those close to somebody with this disorder want to understand why. What can make a person feel such pain or suffer so much that they end up in this rather extreme mindset?

First and foremost it's important to know that this is not a choice. For the people who suffer from BPD, it's not simply a matter of turning it on and off like a light switch. Though an individual may wish that they didn't suffer from their symptoms, it is beyond their control. Therefore

a true understanding of the root cause becomes fundamentally important.

It's Crucial To Understand the Person As a Whole
Sometimes it's a matter of what has gone on within a
family or the environment. Sometimes it's family history
that plays into the individual's likelihood to develop this
condition. It may be something so awful or horrific that
has happened to this person in their life that the BPD becomes their sort of coping mechanism for dealing with it.
The reasons or causes may vary, but the need for help is
common and therefore important.

You need to understand the person as a whole and what
they have been through in their life. Even understanding
family history can help to shed some light on why this
condition may develop. Sometimes there is a very clear
understanding of the presence of this disorder and sometimes it may be a more isolated incident.

Getting to the root cause of what has made the BPD develop is crucial. Not only can it help with diagnosis, but it
can also help with understanding what is going on within
them. Sometimes the feeling of isolation or the severe
self esteem issues may derive from something very serious in nature.

So before we turn our backs on somebody who seems
introverted or socially awkward, it's wise to understand
what be going on within them. Sometimes this sort of behavior is not an escape from being kind or outgoing, but
rather a way of dealing with unfortunate circumstances.
Sometimes all people with BPD want is understanding
and compassion. If they can get that and then receive
diagnosis and treatment, they can live normal lives. So
the causes of BPD become fundamentally important in

allowing an individual to move forward with their life and to cope with what may be lying beneath the surface.

The Most Common Causes That You May Not Anticipate
You may think that you know what causes BPD, but sometimes it's not what it seems. Here we look at the most common root causes which can offer an explanation and hope for a healthy future all at the same time.

- Genetics or family history: This can account for many mental health conditions, and this is no different. Many who have had a family history, particularly within parents, with BPD may experience it in some capacity in their life. It's important to really understand genetics and to know if BPD existed within the family history at all.

- Suffered from trauma or tragedy in life: Those who have suffered through great loss or some adverse circumstances often use symptoms of BPD as a coping mechanism. Something terribly tragic is often too much for somebody to deal with and so they begin to exhibit these symptoms and BPD begins to manifest itself quite easily.

- Childhood abuse or neglect: A very common thread with those who suffer with BPD is the presence of some sort of childhood abuse, neglect, abandonment, or even sexual abuse. This is a very difficult situation as the individual may not have ever properly come to terms with or dealt with this abuse. They may be in denial about what happened and therefore became focused on self loathing, feeling that somehow it was their fault.

- Brain abnormalities: Any sort of chemical imbalance or brain abnormality may cause BPD to develop. This is often unknown to the individual and so they may struggle with what they see as demons their whole life through. This is a difficult one to diagnose and to cope with, but help can be found.

- Other mental health condition present: It is likely that you see mental health conditions coexist together in many cases. It may be as common as depression or something more serious and obscure in nature. Either way you often see more than one mental health condition exist at once, and this may even be what BPD develops out of. This is an instance where the individual really needs some help to cope with daily life as it can be very difficult!

Trying to Accept & Control BPD

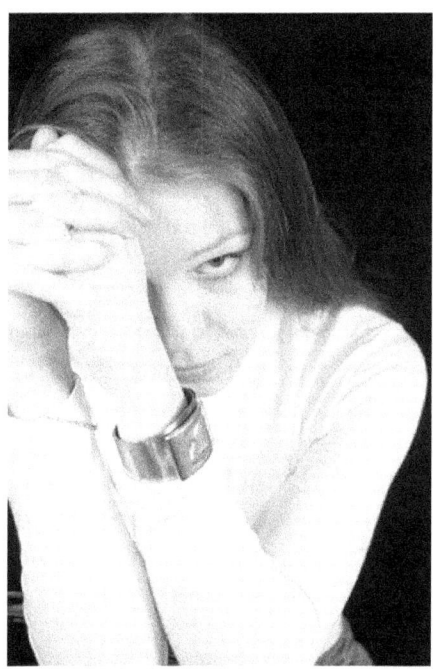

To the outside observer or even the person going through it, the behavior that is associated with Borderline Personality Disorder may be difficult to understand. At times it may seem like depression and at other times it may seem like something as severe as bipolar disorder. The range of emotions and drastic behavior is quite substantial.

Here's the thing that is important to remember, any sort of unusual behavior or wide variances in emotion should be noted. Many people may feel unsure if it is truly BPD, but it's important to look for patterns and triggers that may set the behavior off. Also keeping in tune with the symptoms as noted earlier can be of great help too.

Understanding Even in a Chaotic Situation
BPD can often feel like a very chaotic situation and disorder to live with, for those affected directly by it and for the ones that love them. This is difficult to explain to others outside of it and can make social interactions or just daily life activities seem challenging. It's not a good situation for anybody, but it's important to rise above and learn to make sense of it all.

Obviously diagnosis and treatment are going to be two main components in trying to make sense of it all. Even having the ability to talk to an outside third party or therapist will help to get it out on the table and allow you to move forward. Beyond that though, there may be bigger issues which you may need to try and get ahead of. Being proactive can really help you to rise above the challenges that BPD may present in life.

Here are some things to consider as you try to keep the chaos of BPD based behavior to a minimum:
- Getting to the root cause of the symptoms and behavior: There may very well be something lurking beneath the surface which causes the BPD to come out. There may be something that the individual is in denial about which causes this sometimes erratic behavior to be part of everyday life. Getting to the root cause of the behavior or the issues that plague this person can be of great help. Not only will it help to lessen the BPD behavior, but it will also help to make everyday life so much more enjoyable for all involved.

- Trying to record or keep up with what is happening, when, and what triggers the behavior: Getting in tune with triggers the challenging behavior can be a key element to successfully overcoming it. The behavior is derived from somewhere or something and that's what you need to uncover. You must try to understand if it's stress or anxiety, if it's a specific relationship or dynamic, or if it's just having a bad day that makes this behavior come out in individuals. The triggers can be very telling and allow you to overcome them with practice and treatment.

- Looking for ways to stop the behavior as it happens: This is not easy and it may come with time, but it can be done. Once treatment is received and triggers are identified, then trying to stop the behavior midstream can be very possible. It's important to be patient with this step, but sometimes taking a deep breath and finding a way to gain perspective can be a wonderful way of dealing with things. Stopping the behavior before it gets out of control will be a major element in allowing for a normal life.

- Doing some soul searching to discuss issues that may be difficult to cope with: Trying to get in touch with what causes you distress, anxiety, or difficulties in everyday life can be instrumental. Are you finding it hard to perform in your job? Is there somebody in your life that is causing you great stress? Do you feel that there are changes you can make to help the behavior to stop being so erratic? This takes some very honest soul searching and some changes that may be essential but yet difficult to make and adjust to—but very necessary!

What To Do If You Suspect This Condition In Your Own Life

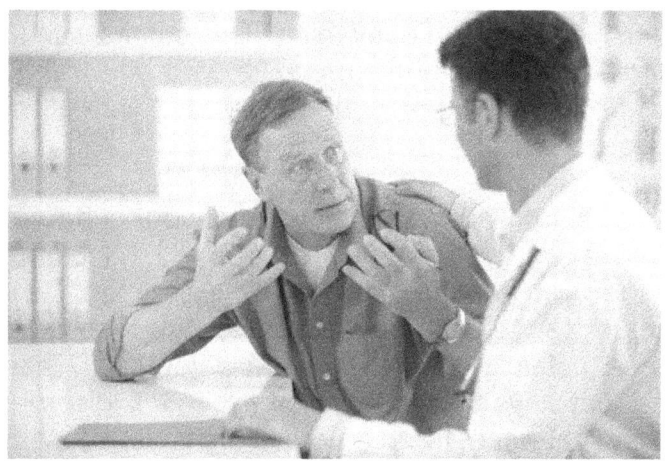

The reality is that BPD can be a very scary thing to come to terms with. There are so many mental health issues and conditions out there, and knowing if you have one can be a bit frightening at times. If you can get in touch with the truth then you can do your part to make living a normal life happen—but it does take strength and honesty with you as an individual!

So what if it's not a loved one that you are worried about, but yourself? What if you are concerned that your behavior has been all over the place and you want to figure out what's going on within you? What if you exhibit several of the symptoms and you are worried that you need to get help, but you aren't quite sure what to do next?

It's a Scary But Very Necessary Step in the Process

To say that it's scary to dig deep and figure out what is going on is an understatement. The truth is that it does take courage to look within yourself and identify the sometimes erratic behavior. To admit that you have extreme self esteem issues or an inability to cope or to form relationships is not an easy thing. This comes with time and a readiness to want to move forward with your life. It can be done, but you must be patient with yourself in the process.

If you really truly suspect that some of your behavior or mannerisms or the way that you cope with things may be BPD, then you need to come to terms with that. It's important to start to keep track of things, and also to talk to the ones that you love and who know you best. There are some great ways to uncover the keys to this disorder and that may mean that living a normal life is very possible again.

If you suspect that BPD is taking over your life, then it's time to get in touch with things. Here are some ways to focus in on the behavior and try to rise above it to get the help that you need:

- Look for patterns and record what goes on within you: This can be the most telling way of discovering what's going on within you. If you can take the time to record your behavior or look for patterns in the way that you feel, it can be of great help. Sometimes elements such as low self esteem may not go away over time, but the difficulty in feeling close to somebody may. When you really take the time to record things and look for patterns, it may also help you to discover triggers for that behavior or to find deep underlying causes for the BPD.

- Start to really analyze any unusual behavior or difficulties in coping with things: Everyone has a bad day, but do you find that your behavior is totally unusual? Do you feel that perhaps things are just not right? Take a step back and gain perspective, both from your point of view and from others as well. If you feel that you can't cope with the everyday occurrences or find that you have difficulties in making it through a day without some sort of unusual behavior, this can help you to get to the path of seeking help that you need.

- Talk to your loved ones to see what they may observe: Sometimes our best cues as to what is really going on, come from those closest to us. Be sure that the friends and family that you ask are close and trusted. Once you know who to ask they may give you more information than you could ever gather yourself. Observations and insight from those closest to you can help you to uncover things that you may not have even realized about yourself. This is an important step in the process!

- Begin to look for help and proper diagnosis: Once you have gathered up your information it's time to get some help. Having the insight to gather the information beforehand is helpful, as a doctor will ask about these elements. Getting a proper diagnosis can happen and so will treatment, but before that you must be honest with yourself and seek out the help that you require. It's not an easy admission, but it's an important one if you wish to move forward with a good and normal life. Take the time to do some research, lean on your loved ones for ideas, and seek out the help that you need to move forward with the diagnosis and then proper treatment. Be your own best advocate and it will go a long way in coping with BPD!

Addressing With a Positive Attitude

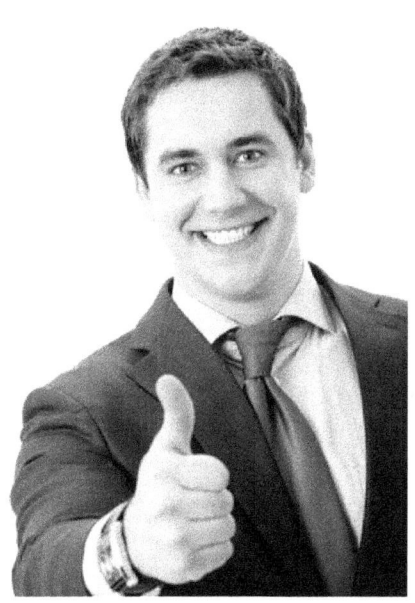

Once you really decide that you believe it is BPD that you are suffering with, then it's time to get some help. This is where you have to learn to speak up for yourself and when you need to put your needs forth in a straightforward and effective manner. If you can have the insight to know that something is amiss and you want to work towards treatment, then it's going to be imperative to speak up for yourself.

This is a point at which you must be open and honest about what you need. It's imperative to be confident about what's working for you and what's not, and that will take some soul searching to determine. If you can really stay focused on the best care for yourself and be ready to figure out what changes must come about, then you have a good shot at normal living again.

Perhaps you have struggled with what you now recognize as Borderline Personality Disorder your entire life. Maybe this is entirely new and therefore taking you off guard as you work through the issues and behavior that are commonly associated with this mental health condition. It doesn't matter how long you have struggled with BPD or how extreme it may be, the point is that you must determine what your needs will be.

This is going to be different for everyone as the severity, frequency, and individual symptoms associated with the condition vary widely. Therefore, it's up to you to take a long hard look at your life and figure out what's working—and more importantly what's not. This isn't always easy and it requires you to be honest, forthcoming, and confident with your choices. Now however is the time to do what works best for you!

Being honest and confident with your choices will lend way to the changes you must make, which we'll get to next. For now though, it's important to first figure out a road to treatment. This journey can be tough to take, but the end result is that you will enjoy a happier and healthier life. That's what it's all about in the end, so it's crucial that you head down this path to a better version of your life.

You can be happy, you can enjoy improved mental health, and you can feel normal again living a life free of symptoms. First you must dig deep to determine what exactly is going on, what is and isn't working for you, and how you move forward to get to the life that you want. This step may take you some time, but it's going to be well worth it in the end when you can minimize your symptoms or get rid of them entirely. Either way this is a step well worth taking and you will feel great clarity when you determine the best way to move forward with your life.

So How Do You Figure It All Out and Move Forward?
The important question is how do you get in touch with that confidence and clarity to know how to move forward? How do you figure out what's best for you and how you proceed with changing things up? How do you incorporate your lifestyle with proper diagnosis and treatment to ensure that you move forward with a life where BPD doesn't rule you? Here are some guidelines to keep in mind and help you to figure things out:

- Putting yourself first and knowing that it's a necessity: This is a time in your life where you must put yourself first. Even if you don't feel good about yourself or have a hard time not putting others first, it's a necessity to put the attention and focus on yourself. This is the only way that you will get what you need and be able to move forward with ease. If you have spent your entire life caring for others or putting your own needs on the back burner, then this may not come easily to you. It's important to know though that putting yourself first will ensure that you can get out of this behavior and into a life that you are happy with.

- Knowing that you are truly worth it: This is another area where people tend to struggle with as major self esteem issues are so strongly associated with Borderline Personality Disorder. You have probably spent a significant time in your life telling yourself that you're not good enough and that you're not worthy or valuable enough. It's time to break the cycle! The only way to move forward with your life in a positive direction is to know that you are worthy of good things and then to get the help that you need—you will be so happy that you did!

- Speaking up for yourself and being your own best advocate: You must be your own best advocate with this disorder, more so than with many other conditions. You must have the insight to see what is working for you in terms of treatment and next steps, and what isn't and needs to be changed. You have to be in tune to how things affect you and then speak up to get the help that you need. Again for a disorder that causes major self esteem issues, it's not always easy to overcome this step, but it's important. If you can get to a place to speak up for your own needs and be the one who looks out for yourself more than any other, then you are handling BPD in a way that will lead towards healing and proper treatment. This will in turn give you major confidence in the process.

- Getting a clear head whenever possible to reflect on how BPD is affecting you and what you can do about it: It's not always easy to take the time to reflect on how BPD is affecting you, but it's necessary. Just as you record the patterns and behaviors and symptoms that grab a hold of your life, you want to keep up with that for the next steps. Know when some form of treatment is work-

36

ing and when you don't feel it's right. Take the time to reflect on how your days are going and how the symptoms are weighing in after a while. Every day may be different, but you must have the ability to get a clear head and analyze what's going on. It won't always be easy, but it will be well worth it if you can enjoy more of your days than suffering through them. Try to think of things that way and it will help you to take the time to reflect.

- Having the courage to recognize that some changes must be made: We are going to get into what changes must be made and how you actually make them next. For now though, as you go through the process of reflection, it's time to get in touch with the fact that the changes must be made. Having the courage to recognize that and reflect upon it will be an important part of your journey. Undoubtedly the disorder has grabbed a hold of your life, perhaps with some traumatic life circumstances. It's time to take it back though. Now is the time to know what's working in your life and what must be changed. Simply having that courage to make the changes and then to actually do the work to get there is all part of healing. It can work, it will work, and you will get your life back— now it's time to do the work to get there and to take your life back and start enjoying it again!

Making Changes In Your Life To Help Life To Feel Normal Again

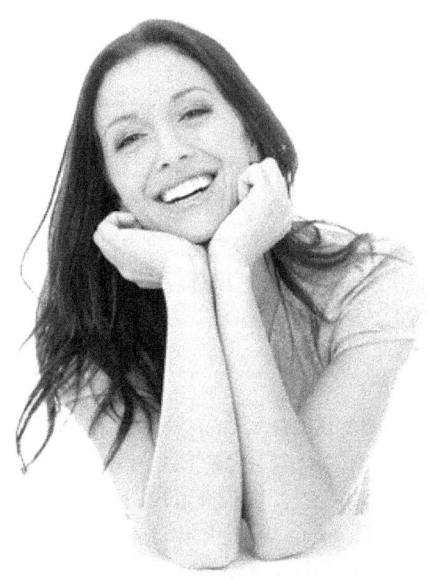

Normal is relative and of course it means different things to different people. To somebody suffering from Border-line Personality Disorder, it can simply mean being able to function in everyday life again. It may mean something as basic as having the ability to develop and maintain re-lationships. Some of the very things that others may take for granted are the elements that people with BPD want in their daily lives.

It's important to have a goal in mind and to stay focused on what's important to you. This is a very individual thing and therefore normalcy is achieved through various methods. Suffice it to say though, that in order to get to that normalcy level, you must be ready to make some changes in your life. Some may be rather significant in nature and some may be a bit more subdued.

Being Prepared To Change Things Up Once and For All Takes Time
This is a very challenging step for many as they work to figure out what's working in their life and what's not. We've already talked about how to evaluate your life and to take a step back to gain perspective. Now it's time to put those observations into real life working order and to take the necessary steps to get to a better life. Sure proper diagnosis and treatment will be a major component within this, but there are also steps that you have to take on your own.

Having the courage to recognize what's working and what's not working takes a certain readiness that not everybody has. You need to be at this step in the process and prepared to do what it takes to move forward with your life. You can do this and you will do this, but you first have to be ready to take the journey. This will eventually lead you to the normalcy that you want and the life that you want to live, but for now it's important to take inventory of what's working, what's not, and what changes you need to make in order to make it all work.

Moving Forward With Important Changes to Achieve True and Lasting Happiness
Again the changes that you make are going to be specific to you and your life, but the point is that you recognize them and then make them. So here we take a look at what sort of things to keep in mind and how you can go about making these critical changes in your life.

- Recognize what's working and most importantly what's not working: We've already discussed the importance of taking inventory in your life. There are bound to be some things that are working quite well, and some for which change is required. Only you know this and therefore honesty is important here! So you must be ready and willing to notice the good things and the bad—and then move forward to getting rid of the elements that may be holding you back.

- Be ready to make some changes that may be rather significant in your life: You may have to change the way that you move throughout your day. You may need to get bad influences or negative people out of your life. You may have to look into the triggers that bring out the undesirable behavior and then move those out for good. This isn't always easy, but this is what will help you to get to normalcy. These changes may be significant and it may be difficult to make them, but the rewards are immeasurable for living with this condition.

- Be able to communicate what you need to change up the things that negatively affect you: Don't be afraid to speak up as to what changes must be made. If it's all about your own good then you have to look out for yourself. You obviously don't want to hurt anybody, but you will never get to the life that you want if you can't speak up for yourself. Be forthcoming in the things that you need to do to make your life more "livable".

- Know that making these changes will help you to get to where you want to be in your life: Be confident in your evaluation and the changes that you make. Know that this path is going to help you to get to the life that you really want. Stay firm in your decisions, speak up for yourself as your best advocate, and be courageous in making the changes needed to allow you to be happy again. You can do this when you are ready and able to make the changes you need in your life once and for all!

Walking On Eggshells: Living With This Condition in a Loved One's Life

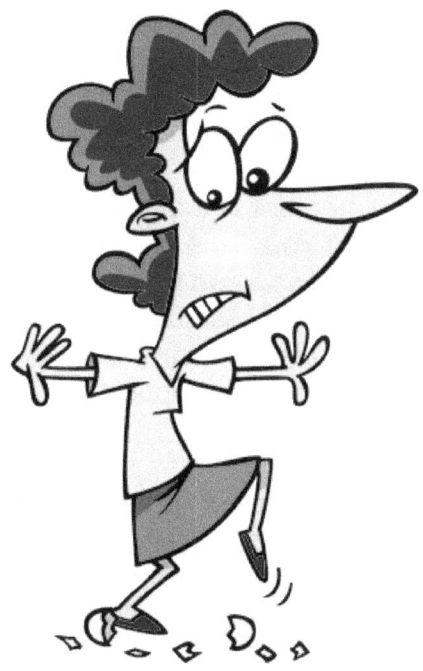

It takes a whole different turn when you look at living with this condition in a loved one's life for that may be much more difficult in some situations. Though the person who suffers from BPD is the one that so much attention is focused on, the truth is that the person who loves and lives with them has much to contend with as well. So it's important to note this and to provide some help to the loved ones of an individual suffering from Borderline Personality Disorder.

It's completely natural but unfortunate, that the loved ones of somebody who suffers from BPD are often forgotten about. Though they may not be dealing with the disease directly, it is certainly a very big part of their life.

There is Help and Relief for Both of You
The truth is that providing the care and compassion that their loved one may need can sometimes feel like a full time job. It is therefore quite important to put forth thought and a plan for the people who love the person suffering from this challenging disorder.

What you must remember is that there is help, not only for them, but also for you. This is a treatable condition and it can be one that you can both live with, but there must be a certain readiness in taking the necessary steps to move forward. You can't force this upon your loved one, but can only be there to support them through the ups and downs.

There is no doubt that this can be challenging and frustrating to live with, for both you and them, but it will also be something that you can move forward with if the right treatment is sought out. When that happens, you will be able to enjoy life together and that can hopefully bring about some relief.

This is a difficult medical condition, but the good news is that so much more is known about it now than there ever used to be. There are ways to get help to those who need it and simply understanding it is possible. There is a light at the end of the tunnel—for both them and you, so know that as you move forward in caring for and supporting your loved one!

Give Yourself Time and Attention to Provide Them With the Support That They Need
This disorder is of course, very much about them, but it's also about you. To love somebody with Borderline Per-

sonality Disorder sometimes takes patience, dedication, and loyalty, particularly when times get tough. Know that having an outlet to feel frustrated is healthy and natural, and the rest will fall into place. Here are some ideas to help you to cope and to be there for your loved one in the process.

- Support your loved one in this important journey: This is a challenging journey for both of you. What your loved one needs more than anything else is your support. This may come easily at some times and not at others, but the point is that you provide it. They may even resist your support at times, but know that it's going to help them in the long run. Be patient and be ready to support them as they walk through this journey and hopefully move towards the treatment that they need.

- Have an outlet for you to feel frustrated and be human: It's okay to feel frustrated and to doubt yourself or even your relationship at times. So long as you don't feel this way or verbalize it in front of them, you are doing fine. You do need an outlet to get that frustration out, whether it's therapy or some sort of healthy and safe environment to be able to vent. You are human and you need to allow yourself to feel that way, so get out the frustration that you feel. If you have that healthy and happy outlet then you have a far better chance of being able to be there for your loved one to give them the support that they need.

- Be patient and compassionate, but also be honest and straightforward with your loved one: Be there for them and try your best to be empathetic and compassionate about what they are going through. It's not always easy and you must recognize that, but you love this person and want to help them. If you have your outlet then it makes being compassionate and patient so much easier. Take the time to understand what they feel and be honest with them whenever necessary. This will help them and allow them to see the situation and the disorder for what it is in both of your lives.

- Know what you can do to help and what must come from the individual directly: Be there to support them, but also know that you can't force anything either. If you want to make it work, then you must allow them to make changes. You can support them and help them along the way, but wanting to move forward and make important changes must come from them directly. Just be aware of that and never force things—let them take their own course through their actions and choices.

Helping a Child To Cope With Early Symptoms & Protecting Children From BPD Behavior

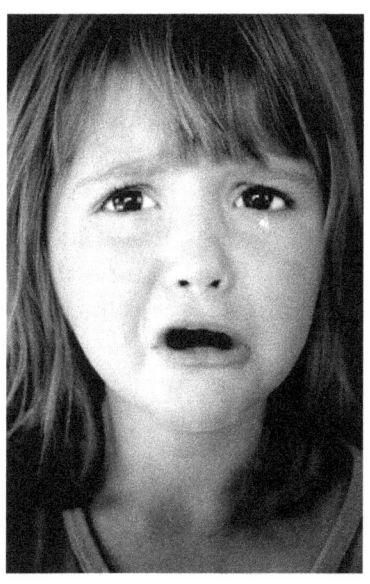

You never want to see your own child suffer, and you certainly never want them to have any sort of health problem. Though they aren't often recognized as readily as actual health problems, the truth is that mental health conditions such as Borderline Personality Disorder can be just as challenging as physical health problems. Not only does a child not know how to cope with this sort of thing, but kids can be cruel and make fun of them for the troubling behavior that is their norm.

As a parent you want to be in tune to the early symptoms. You also want to keep a keen eye on your child if BPD runs in the family at all. If somebody in your immediate family has suffered with BPD, then you want to be sure that you are aware of this in your child. The symptoms may be a bit more subtle at first and could easily be confused with temper tantrums or other similar behavior. Therefore it's up to you as the parent to see what you can do to help them—and the earlier the better!

You Can Help Your Child and You Will Work Through It Together
If your child already suffers from this disorder, know that there is help to be found. You need not beat yourself up for not noticing the signs earlier, but just get your child the help that they need when you can. This is absolutely something that you can find treatment for, particularly with kids, so know that help is on the way.

Equally as important for your child is to help protect them when a family member or loved one has BPD. Sometimes the behavior exhibited can be disturbing, challenging, and even scary to a child. Be there to help them through and try to explain things in simple to understand terms. If your child knows that they can count on you through this type of situation, then it will make for a much more livable situation.

Here are some helpful tips to keep in mind to help your child live with BPD in any capacity, and to help them to enjoy a normal life.

- Be proactive enough to recognize the early symptoms: Now that you see what the symptoms and signs of BPD are, you can be proactive as a parent. If you start to notice unusual changes or symptoms, then be ready to get them some help or at least get them evaluated. This may be what helps them to live a normal life and you can be the

48

key to it. Awareness and the ability to act on getting proper diagnosis and treatment if you suspect BPD is crucial!

- Try to protect them from the BPD behavior of others when applicable: It may not be your child that you are worried about directly, but a loved one. If that's the case then do your best to shield your child from the sometimes frustrating or even scary behavior that BPD can bring about. Be honest with them and talk about the disorder in appropriate terms. Help them to not feel afraid and to always be there to support them if a loved one suffers from this. You are their best support in this situation!

- Try to help them in coping with their own potential for BPD driven behavior: Don't ever point fingers, but do begin to help them to see when certain behavior is not necessarily the norm. The honesty will help them to come to terms with things much easier, and will allow you to provide them the help that they need. Coping is a big part of the equation for kids who suffer from BPD. The good news is that diagnosis and treatment can really help to lessen the effects and provide normalcy, particularly for children.

- Be in tune to what your child may be going through: Know that it may be tough to be a child with BPD and be there for them. Get them the help that they need sooner rather than later, and try not to give into the trap of giving it time and waiting to see what happens. Be ready to jump into action if something just doesn't feel right, even if it's simply to get to a therapist first and foremost. Know that kids can sometimes be cruel too and if they are exhibiting such behavior at school or with other kids as they are with you, then it may be a very difficult road for them. Be supportive, compassionate, sympathetic, and get them the help that they need quickly to help with their daily lives.

- Treat BPD in a child differently than in an adult—they may not know how to deal with it: An adult needs to ask for help, but a child may not know how to do that. They may not be aware that their behavior is not the norm and so it's up to you to help them see this. Don't take a hands off approach with kids as they really need you to help them through the challenges that this disorder can present. Be supportive to them in an entirely different way that takes control of the situation and sees them through to treatment. Help them to normalcy as soon as possible and be their best advocate. This is a totally different approach than you would use with an adult, but it's a necessary one as kids need you to depend on in this situation!

Is What They Say True—Can You Believe the Myths?

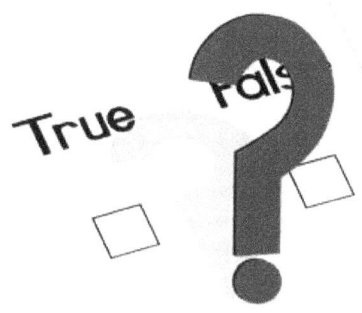

The biggest problem with Borderline Personality Disorder is that it is so grossly misunderstood. The good news is that there is a lot more information out there than ever before and therefore proper diagnosis and treatment is possible and likely. The bad news however is that the mainstream doesn't really understand what this health condition is all about.

It's important to note that there are a lot of myths out there about BPD, none of which are true. It's also imperative that the people who suffer from this condition never for a moment think that it's their fault. Part of that is education and learning to debunk the myths that surround this condition. Therefore, simply bringing these myths to life and allowing people to see what others may believe without being educated can be helpful.

Dispelling the Myths is an Important Part of the Education Process
The myths can be hurtful, particularly because they center around this being a condition that people choose to have. Not only that, but some believe that this is simply about behavior and personality rather than mental illness. Anybody who suffers from BPD or who loves somebody who does, knows that this is a medical condition just like anything else. So seeing the myths out there can be a great way of moving forward and recognizing that help is truly needed.

Here we look at some of the most common myths surrounding BPD, and the notable part is that they are mostly ridiculous and no factual basis lies within them. These myths are derived out of fear and out of a lack of education. Though they may be hurtful, it's important to know that they are not true and to be part of the education process. Often times, people fear the very things that they don't understand, and that's what these myths are all about.

BPD is quickly becoming a disorder for which people understand and through time and education in the mainstream, these myths will go away. For now though, it's important to recognize that they exist and to work through them together. Never let these slow down your progress or inhibit your ability to move forward. Simply recognize that they are out there and then find a way to move past them and use them as motivation to move forward with your life once and for all.

The Most Common Myths Surrounding Borderline Personality Disorder

1. People with Borderline Personality Disorder are simply seeking out attention: Clearly nobody would want the attention that comes along with this disorder. The attention that somebody who has BPD receives is mostly negative and therefore it's ridiculous that anybody would seek this out. Clearly this comes from a lack of education as the behavior is often out of the person's control and therefore disruptive to their everyday life. This must never be taken seriously as anybody who knows or truly understands BPD would recognize that this makes no sense.

2. This is not a real disorder, but rather something that the individual can control: Since the word "borderline" exists as part of the description, people tend to cast this aside as a real disorder. This is a very real, legitimate, and founded mental health condition for which people need help with to function in everyday life. Just because this isn't necessarily as extreme as other mental illnesses, doesn't mean that it's not to be taken seriously. This comes from people who may have heard a little bit about this condition, but who don't really understand the implications of it.

3. The people with this condition are introverts with low self esteem to begin with: Though there may be introverted behavior, these are not people that want to be completely detached from anything or anyone else. The low self esteem may be part of the condition or may be from some other tragedy that the individual has suffered from in their lives.

Neither low self esteem or an introverted nature is anything to be ashamed with. Though they can be associated with this disorder, it doesn't mean that this sort of behavior or thought process can't be reversed—treatment can be a helpful step towards achieving normalcy!

4. This is a condition that is not treatable and therefore healing must come from within: This may be the most ridiculous myth of all for treatment is undoubtedly available for those that need it. Though the form of treatment may vary, the availability of it is definitely there for the taking. It's important to recognize this and to know that this is a legitimate mental health condition for which treatment is surely available—life can be normal and worthwhile to enjoy again!

Learning to Live With BPD and Making It Part of Everyday Life

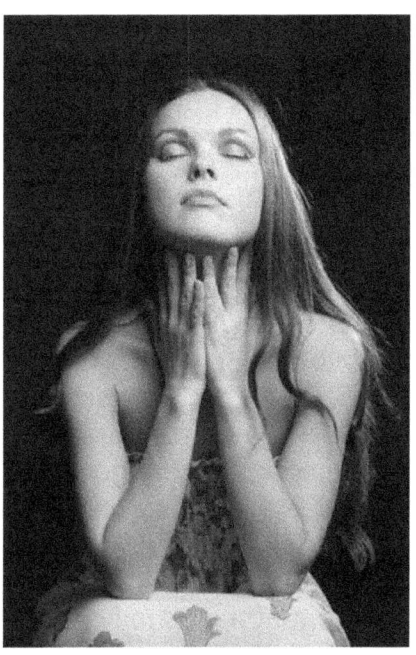

You've seen first hand that Borderline Personality Disorder can be a frustrating disorder, but it doesn't have to rule your life. The reality is that you can make this condition work for you and achieve the normalcy that you've been searching for. That comes as great news to those who suffer from it and the people who love them.

You've seen that much of the ability to live with this condition comes from making important changes in life that will allow you to be happy. You have also seen that you need to figure out what's working and what's not working so that you can create the environment that lifts you up rather than drags you down. If you can stay focused on these elements, you have a great chance of taking your life back.

As you make these big moves in your life, you also want to be sure to stay focused on your long term happiness. You need to keep a clear head, be diligent with your treatment plan, and always put yourself first. The more information comes out about BPD, the more people will have a good chance of enjoying a healthy and wonderful life that centers around happiness and not the disorder ruling them.

The reality is that once diagnosis happens and a proper treatment comes into play, you will be able to move forward with things. This can be very reassuring while also recognizing that there is a certain amount of courage required to make the important changes. You can do it and you will do it and you will have a wonderful life awaiting you!

Here are some important things to keep in mind as you focus on taking control of your life and ensuring that Borderline Personality Disorder doesn't rule you.

- Finding a mix and balance that works best for you: The routine that you get into and the way that you live with this disorder may vary from others. Just as the symptoms and severity vary amongst individuals, so too does the way that people can cope with it in their lives. You need to find the balance, the routine, and the plan moving forward that works for you. This takes time, diligence, and the ability to put yourself and your needs first. Once you find that and you create that balance, you will know it. You will then learn to move forward in a way that ensures pure and lasting happiness!

- Determining a treatment plan that will fit into your life and allow you to feel happy and normal again: Once you get diagnosed and start to work with a medical professional that understands your needs, this will be a great beginning. Fitting that treatment plan into your life and making it work for your lifestyle is an important step. You need to know that you can feel happy and normal again, and your treatment should accompany and enable that. It's supposed to go hand in hand, so be sure that this is what truly happens.

- Knowing your triggers and avoiding the elements that can contribute to BPD behavior coming back again: If you've taken the time to reflect then you know first hand what may set off the BPD behavior and issues. If you are aware of that then you can by all means avoid the triggers that contribute to your symptoms. Avoiding these elements, limiting your exposure, and making positive changes are all what will help you to live with BPD—and never let it rule your life again!

- Finding the things that make you happy and focusing on them moving forward: Part of this is focusing on what makes you truly happy, because that's an important aspect of treatment as well. Think of the people and things that bring you happiness and then integrate them into your life in a cohesive manner. This will help you to make positive change and to actually enjoy your life for a change. That's ultimately what it's all about, with or without BPD, it's about finding what makes you happy and then focusing on this moving forward.

Conclusion

Borderline Personality Disorder is a very common condition that has long been misunderstood. Though you may have been concerned before, now you know that this is a very treatable condition that you can live with in a perfectly normal way. In the past not as much was known or understood about this disorder, but now it has become a very well understood medical condition that there is great help for.

It's important to recognize the symptoms and to know what warrants asking for help. Though BPD can be confused with other mental health issues, there are some signs and symptoms that are very closely linked. Be in tune to what is going on, look for patterns, and know when to ask for help. This may seem obvious, but sometimes education such as you have now can be what helps you in the long run.

The right medical professional who truly understands this condition can be of great help. They can help to get you proper diagnosis and then figure out a treatment plan that works for you. It's always important to be your own best advocate though, so be certain that you get the time to speak up and do what works best for you. If something isn't working, then find another avenue.

You don't have to let Borderline Personality Disorder rule your life anymore—you can take control over things! If you can take a look at your life and figure out what's working and what's not, then that's a great start. If you can find the courage to make the important changes that will allow you to enjoy your life and get away from the negative aspects and triggers, then that will make a huge impact.

You can live with BPD and enjoy normalcy, you can take back your life and find the things that make you happy. There is great treatment and help that will allow you to be happy and to enjoy the person that you are, as well as the life that you create. Be aware of what BPD is, how it manifests itself, and get in touch with everything you feel. Then it's all about getting back to enjoying life and creating true and ultimate happiness for yourself! Thank you for reading and good luck!